The Drive of Rory McIlroy

THE DRIVE OF RORY McILROY:

A Golfing Legend

Daniel T. Nelson

The Drive of Rory McIlroy

All rights reserved. No part of this book may be reproduced, stored in a retrieval system, or transmitted in any form or by any means, electronic, mechanical, photocopying, recording, or otherwise, without the prior written permission of the publisher, except in the case of brief quotations embodied in critical articles and reviews.

Copyright © 2024 by [Daniel T. Nelson]

The Drive of Rory McIlroy

TABLE OF CONTENTS

INTRODUCTION

CHAPTER 1: THE EARLY YEARS :

1.1: A Childhood Passion for Golf

1.2: Introduction to the Sport

1.3: Early Influences and Inspiration

CHAPTER 2: THE RISING TALENT

2.1: Emerging as a Junior Golfer

2.2: Amateur Successes and Milestones

2.3: Decision to Turn Professional

CHAPTER 3: THE JOURNEY TO STARDOM:

3.1: Early Professional Career Challenges

3.2: Breakthrough Wins and Notable Performances

3.3: Establishing a Name on the PGA Tour

CHAPTER 4: MAJOR TRIUMPH

The Drive of Rory McIlroy

4.1:The Quest for Major Championship

4.2:The 2011 U.S. Open Victory

4.3: Masters, Open Championships, and PGA Championship Successes

CHAPTER 5: THE MENTAL GAME

5.1: Mental Toughness and Resilience

5.2:Overcoming Setbacks and Challenges

5.3:Mindset and Approach to Pressure Situations

CHAPTER 6: TECHNIQUES AND TRAINING

6.1:The Evolution of Rory McIlroy's Swing

6.2:Training Regimens and Fitness Routines

6.3: Collaborations with Coaches and Experts

CHAPTER 7: OFF THE COURSE

7.1:Personal Life and Interests

7.2:Charitable Endeavours and Giving Back

7.3:Balancing Fame and Privacy

CHAPTER 8: RIVALRIES AND RELATIONSHIPS

The Drive of Rory McIlroy

8.1: Rory McIlroy: Competing Against Golf's Elite

8.2: Friendships and Camaraderie on Tour

8.3: Legacy and Impact on the Sport

CHAPTER 9: THE FUTURE OF RORY MCILROY

9.1: Charting a Course of Ambition and Aspiration

9.2: Continuing to Push the Boundaries and Redefining Greatness

9.3: Legacy Beyond the Fairways

CHAPTER 10: REFLECTIONS AND LESSONS

10.1: Inspirational Insights for Golfers and Fans Alike

CONCLUSION:

The Drive of Rory McIlroy

INTRODUCTION

In the hushed reverence of a golf course, where the whisper of a breeze and the thud of a perfectly struck ball resonate like poetry, one man's name echoes with a resonance that transcends the sport itself: Rory McIlroy. His story is not just one of a golfing prodigy, but a saga of relentless determination, unwavering passion, and an insatiable hunger for greatness.

Born in the lush green landscapes of Hollywood, Northern Ireland, on May 4, 1989, Rory McIlroy's

The Drive of Rory McIlroy

journey to the summit of golfing immortality began with a childhood dream and a singular obsession: mastering the art of the swing. From the moment he first gripped a club, there was an undeniable sense of destiny coursing through his veins, propelling him forward on a path paved with ambition and boundless potential.

But it was on the windswept fairways of his homeland that McIlroy's talent truly blossomed, honed by the raw beauty of the Irish countryside and the fierce competition of local tournaments. With each swing and each putt, he etched his name into the annals of golfing lore, his precocious talent drawing comparisons to the legends who had come before him.

Yet, for all his natural gifts, it was McIlroy's unyielding drive and relentless work ethic that set him apart. In the crucible of competition, he thrived, his steely resolve and unshakable focus propelling him to heights few could have imagined. From his maiden victory at the 2009 Dubai Desert Classic to his record-breaking triumphs at the U.S. Open, Open Championship, and PGA Championship, McIlroy's journey was defined by a singular pursuit: the relentless quest for perfection.

The Drive of Rory McIlroy

But beyond the glitz and glamour of the major championships, McIlroy's legacy extends far beyond the confines of the golf course. Through his tireless efforts to grow the game and his unwavering commitment to philanthropy, he has become not just a sporting icon but a global ambassador for the power of perseverance and the boundless potential of the human spirit.

As we embark on this journey through the life and career of Rory McIlroy, we bear witness to the triumphs and tribulations of a true sporting legend. Through the highs and lows, the victories and defeats, one thing remains constant: the unwavering drive of a man who dared to dream the impossible, and in doing so, forever altered the landscape of golf history.

CHAPTER 1: THE EARLY YEARS :

Rory McIlroy, a name synonymous with excellence in golf, didn't rise to prominence overnight. His journey to becoming one of the sport's most celebrated figures was marked by passion, determination, and unwavering dedication. In this exploration of McIlroy's early years, we delve into the formative experiences and driving forces that shaped him into the golfing legend he is today.

The Drive of Rory McIlroy

Early Beginnings:

Born on May 4, 1989, in Hollywood, Northern Ireland, Rory McIlroy's affinity for golf was evident from a tender age. His father, Gerry McIlroy, introduced him to the sport at the age of just two, fashioning makeshift clubs out of plastic. By the age of seven, Rory was already showcasing exceptional talent on the golf course, impressing seasoned players and coaches alike with his natural swing and remarkable composure.

Nurturing Talent:

Recognising Recognising Recognising his son's potential, Gerry McIlroy invested countless hours into Rory's development, serving as his coach, mentor, and biggest supporter. Under his father's guidance, Rory honed his skills at the Holywood Golf Club, where he quickly rose through the ranks, setting numerous course records and winning junior championships with remarkable ease. This early exposure to competition instilled in Rory a fierce competitive spirit and an insatiable hunger for success.

The Drive of Rory McIlroy

Rise to Prominence:

As Rory's reputation as a prodigious talent continued to grow, so did his ambitions. At the age of 15, he caught the attention of the golfing world by winning the prestigious West of Ireland Championship, becoming the youngest-ever winner of the event. His meteoric rise continued unabated, culminating in victory at the 2006 European Amateur Championship, a feat that solidified his status as one of golf's brightest prospects.

Turning Professional:

In 2007, at the age of 18, Rory McIlroy made the pivotal decision to turn professional, a move that would alter the course of his career forever. Armed with unparalleled talent and unwavering self-belief, he wasted no time in making his mark on the professional circuit, earning his European Tour card and securing his first victory at the Dubai Desert Classic in 2009. With each triumph, McIlroy's legend continued to grow, captivating audiences around the globe with his electrifying play and magnetic charisma.

The Drive for Greatness:

The Drive of Rory McIlroy

What sets Rory McIlroy apart from his peers is not just his exceptional talent but also his insatiable drive for greatness. Behind the effortless swings and flawless putts lies a relentless work ethic and an unyielding desire to push the boundaries of his own potential. Whether it's grinding on the practice range until dusk or meticulously analysing every aspect of his game, McIlroy's commitment to excellence knows no bounds.

Legacy and Impact:

Today, Rory McIlroy stands as one of golf's most iconic figures, with an illustrious career that includes four major championships, countless tour victories, and a legacy that transcends the sport itself. Beyond his on-course achievements, McIlroy's impact extends far beyond the fairways, inspiring a new generation of golfers and captivating fans with his humility, sportsmanship, and philanthropy.

From his humble beginnings in Holywood to his ascent to the pinnacle of golfing glory, Rory McIlroy's journey is a testament to the power of passion, perseverance, and unwavering dedication. As he continues to etch his name into the annals of golfing history, one thing remains abundantly clear: the drive of Rory McIlroy knows no bounds.

1.1: A Childhood Passion for Golf

Rory McIlroy's journey into the world of golf began at a remarkably young age, fueled by an innate passion and unwavering determination. Born on May 4, 1989, in Hollywood, Northern Ireland, McIlroy was practically destined for greatness on the greens. His childhood was steeped in the sport, with both his parents, Gerry and Rosie, fostering his love for golf from the tender age of two.

Under the guidance of his father, who worked multiple jobs to support his son's budding talent, McIlroy honed his skills at the Holywood Golf Club, where he quickly became a prodigious young talent. His dedication and natural aptitude for the game were evident to all who witnessed his effortless swing and unwavering focus on the course.

Despite his young age, McIlroy exhibited maturity and determination beyond his years, spending countless hours practising his game and fine-tuning his technique.

The Drive of Rory McIlroy

His commitment to excellence was unwavering, and his passion for golf only intensified with each passing day.

McIlroy's breakthrough moment came at the age of nine, when he recorded a remarkable score of 40 for nine holes at his home club, a feat that left seasoned golfers astounded and served as a testament to his prodigious talent. From that moment on, it was clear that McIlroy was destined for greatness in the world of golf.

As he continued to progress through his formative years, McIlroy's reputation as a rising star in the golfing world continued to grow. He represented Ireland in various amateur competitions, showcasing his exceptional skill and unwavering determination on the international stage.

McIlroy's childhood passion for golf was not solely driven by a desire for personal success but also by a deep-seated love for the sport itself. He found solace and joy on the golf course, relishing the challenge of each new round and the opportunity to push himself to new heights.

Throughout his childhood, McIlroy remained grounded and humble, never losing sight of the values instilled in him by his parents and mentors. His commitment to his craft and his unwavering dedication to excellence served as inspiration to aspiring golfers around the world, proving that with passion, perseverance, and a love for the game, anything is possible.

In essence, Rory McIlroy's childhood passion for golf was not just a hobby or pastime but rather a calling that would ultimately propel him to the pinnacle of the sport. From his earliest days on the greens of Holywood to his triumphs on the world stage, McIlroy's journey serves as a testament to the transformative power of passion, dedication, and unwavering belief in oneself.

1.2: Introduction to the Sport

Rory McIlroy's introduction to the sport of golf was a serendipitous moment that would ultimately shape the trajectory of his life and career. Born into a family with a deep appreciation for the game, McIlroy's journey began at the tender age of two, when he first picked up a golf club under the watchful eye of his father, Gerry.

Growing up in Holywood, Northern Ireland, McIlroy was surrounded by the lush green fairways of the Holywood Golf Club, where his father worked multiple jobs to support his son's burgeoning passion for the sport. It was here, amidst the rolling hills and pristine greens, that McIlroy discovered his love for golf and

The Drive of Rory McIlroy

embarked on a journey that would see him rise to become one of the greatest players of his generation.

From his earliest days on the course, McIlroy displayed an uncanny talent and a natural affinity for the game. His swing was effortless, his focus unwavering, and his determination palpable. Despite his young age, McIlroy approached each round with the poise and maturity of a seasoned professional, displaying a level of skill and composure far beyond his years.

As McIlroy's passion for golf continued to grow, so too did his drive to excel in the sport. He dedicated countless hours to practicing his game, tirelessly honing his skills and perfecting his technique. His commitment to his craft was unmatched, and he embraced the challenges of the game with a tenacity and resilience that set him apart from his peers.

McIlroy's introduction to golf was not just a casual interest or hobby, but rather a calling that would consume him entirely. He found solace and purpose on the course, relishing the opportunity to challenge himself and push the boundaries of his abilities. Golf became more than just a sport to McIlroy—it was a way of life, a passion that fueled his every waking moment.

The Drive of Rory McIlroy

As McIlroy's reputation as a rising star in the golfing world grew, so too did his drive to succeed. He set his sights on the highest echelons of the sport, driven by a relentless pursuit of greatness and an unwavering belief in his own abilities. With each passing tournament and every milestone achieved, McIlroy's drive only intensified, propelling him ever closer to his ultimate goal of becoming a golfing legend.

Rory McIlroy's introduction to the sport of golf was not merely a chance encounter but rather the beginning of a lifelong journey marked by passion, dedication, and an unyielding drive to succeed. From his humble beginnings on the greens of Holywood to his triumphs on the world stage, McIlroy's story serves as a testament to the transformative power of perseverance, determination, and an unwavering belief in oneself.

1.3: Early Influences and Inspiration

Rory McIlroy's early influences and sources of inspiration played a pivotal role in shaping his drive and determination to become a golfing legend. From the

The Drive of Rory McIlroy

supportive guidance of his family to the inspiration he drew from golfing icons, McIlroy's journey to greatness was fueled by a rich tapestry of influences that left an indelible mark on his life and career.

At the heart of McIlroy's early influences was his family, particularly his father, Gerry, whose unwavering support and dedication to his son's passion for golf served as a cornerstone of McIlroy's journey. From the moment McIlroy first picked up a golf club at the age of two, Gerry recognised his son's natural talent and made it his mission to nurture and cultivate that potential. He worked multiple jobs to afford McIlroy the opportunity to pursue his passion, sacrificing his own time and resources to ensure that his son had every chance to succeed.

In addition to his family, McIlroy drew inspiration from the rich history and tradition of golf itself, finding motivation in the exploits of legendary players who had come before him. He idolised the likes of Jack Nicklaus, Tiger Woods, and Seve Ballesteros, studying their games and emulating their techniques in his own quest for excellence. Their achievements served as a constant reminder to McIlroy of the heights that could be reached

The Drive of Rory McIlroy

through hard work, dedication, and an unwavering belief in oneself.

McIlroy's early influences extended beyond the confines of the golf course, with his upbringing in Northern Ireland instilling in him a strong sense of resilience and determination. Growing up amidst the backdrop of the Troubles, McIlroy witnessed firsthand the power of perseverance in the face of adversity, an experience that would later shape his approach to overcoming challenges both on and off the course.

As McIlroy's career began to take shape, he continued to draw inspiration from those around him, surrounding himself with a team of coaches, mentors, and advisors who helped guide and support him on his journey. Their collective wisdom and expertise provided McIlroy with the tools he needed to refine his game and navigate the complexities of professional golf, while their unwavering belief in his abilities served as a constant source of motivation and encouragement.

Rory McIlroy's early influences and sources of inspiration were instrumental in fueling his drive and determination to become a golfing legend. From the unwavering support of his family to the rich tradition of the sport itself, McIlroy's journey was shaped by a myriad of factors that ultimately propelled him to the pinnacle of the golfing world.

CHAPTER 2:THE RISING TALENT

In the illustrious realm of professional golf, few names resonate with the same level of admiration and awe as Rory McIlroy. From his early days as a prodigious talent in Northern Ireland to his ascent to the summit of the golfing world, McIlroy's journey is a testament to unwavering dedication, raw talent, and an unyielding drive for excellence. This article delves into the remarkable rise of Rory McIlroy, tracing his path from a young boy with a dream to one of the most dominant forces in the sport today.

The Drive of Rory McIlroy

Early Years and Beginnings:

Born on May 4, 1989, in Holywood, Northern Ireland, Rory McIlroy showed a natural affinity for golf from a tender age. Introduced to the game by his father, Gerry, who worked multiple jobs to support his son's burgeoning passion, McIlroy quickly displayed an extraordinary aptitude for the sport. By the age of seven, he was already hitting 40-yard drives, foreshadowing the remarkable power and precision that would define his game in the years to come.

Rise Through the Ranks:

McIlroy's ascent through the ranks of junior and amateur golf was meteoric. He captured his first significant victory at the age of nine, winning the World Championship for his age group. As he progressed through his teenage years, McIlroy continued to amass trophies and accolades, showcasing a level of talent that belied his young age. His breakthrough on the international stage came in 2007, when he secured the prestigious silver medal as the leading amateur at the Open Championship.

The Drive of Rory McIlroy

Professional Success and Major Victories:

In 2007, McIlroy made the transition to professional golf, and it didn't take long for him to make his mark. He secured his first professional win at the 2009 Dubai Desert Classic, setting the stage for a career defined by dominance and consistency. McIlroy's crowning moment came in 2011, when he claimed his first major championship victory at the U.S. Open, becoming the youngest winner of the tournament since 1923. This triumph served as a harbinger of greater things to come, as McIlroy went on to capture three more major titles, including the PGA Championship in 2012 and 2014, as well as the Open Championship in 2014.

Mental Strength and Resilience:

Beyond his prodigious physical talents, Rory McIlroy's success can also be attributed to his exceptional mental fortitude and resilience. In the face of adversity and setbacks, he has consistently demonstrated an ability to bounce back stronger, using disappointments as fuel for future triumphs. Whether it's overcoming final-round collapses or battling through injuries, McIlroy's unwavering belief in his abilities has propelled him to greater heights time and time again.

The Drive of Rory McIlroy

Legacy and Impact:

As Rory McIlroy continues to etch his name into the annals of golfing history, his impact on the sport extends far beyond his impressive trophy haul. Through his philanthropic endeavours, including the establishment of the Rory Foundation, he has used his platform to make a positive difference in the lives of others, embodying the values of sportsmanship and giving back. Moreover, his charismatic personality and engaging demeanour have endeared him to fans around the globe, ensuring that his legacy will endure for generations to come.

In the pantheon of golfing legends, Rory McIlroy's name shines brightly as a testament to the power of talent, determination, and perseverance. From his humble beginnings in Northern Ireland to his status as one of the most recognisable figures in the world of sports, McIlroy's journey is a testament to the transformative power of the game of golf. As he continues to chase new heights and inspire future generations, one thing remains certain: the drive of Rory McIlroy is an enduring force that will continue to shape the world of golf for years to come.

The Drive of Rory McIlroy

2.1: Emerging as a Junior Golfer

In the realm of golfing greatness, Rory McIlroy's journey from junior prodigy to professional powerhouse is nothing short of inspirational. From swinging his first club as a toddler to conquering the world's most prestigious courses, McIlroy's rise is a testament to talent, determination, and unwavering passion for the game.

McIlroy's introduction to golf came at an early age, growing up in Holywood, Northern Ireland. Encouraged by his father, Gerry, himself an accomplished player, Rory's affinity for the sport was evident from the start. By the age of 8, he was already making waves on the local circuit, showcasing a natural flair for the game that belied his tender years.

As a junior golfer, McIlroy's potential was undeniable. His dedication to honing his skills saw him spend countless hours on the practice range, refining his swing, and sharpening his short game. Blessed with exceptional

The Drive of Rory McIlroy

talent and an insatiable appetite for success, he quickly emerged as one of the most promising young talents in the world of golf.

McIlroy's breakthrough came in 2004 when, at just 15 years old, he won the prestigious West of Ireland Championship, becoming the youngest-ever winner of the event. This victory served as a harbinger of things to come, as McIlroy continued to dominate the amateur circuit, claiming titles and breaking records with remarkable regularity.

But it was his triumph at the 2007 European Amateur Championship that truly announced McIlroy's arrival on the global stage. With a flawless display of skill and composure, he cruised to victory, capturing the imagination of golf fans around the world and solidifying his status as one of the sport's brightest prospects.

By the time McIlroy turned professional in 2007, he was already a household name in golfing circles. His seamless transition to the pro ranks was marked by a string of impressive performances, including his maiden

The Drive of Rory McIlroy

European Tour victory at the 2009 Dubai Desert Classic. From there, McIlroy's ascent was meteoric, as he went on to claim multiple major championships, including the coveted Masters, U.S. Open, The Open Championship, and PGA Championship.

Today, Rory McIlroy stands as one of the most accomplished and beloved figures in the history of golf. His journey from junior sensation to global superstar serves as a source of inspiration for aspiring golfers everywhere, reminding us all that with talent, hard work, and unwavering determination, anything is possible on the fairways of life.

2.2: Amateur Successes and Milestones

Rory McIlroy, a name synonymous with golfing greatness, began his journey to stardom as a prodigious amateur golfer. His early successes and milestones laid the foundation for a remarkable professional career that would follow.

The Drive of Rory McIlroy

McIlroy's rise to prominence in the amateur ranks was nothing short of spectacular. Hailing from Northern Ireland, he showcased his immense talent from a young age, capturing the attention of the golfing world with his exceptional skill and natural ability.

One of McIlroy's earliest triumphs came in 2006, when he won the European Amateur Championship at the tender age of 17. This victory signalled the beginning of what would be a string of impressive achievements on the amateur circuit.

In 2007, McIlroy continued to solidify his status as a rising star by winning the prestigious West of Ireland Championship and the Irish Amateur Championship in the same year. These victories highlighted his dominance on both the national and international stages and earned him widespread recognition as one of the most promising talents in the game.

However, it was McIlroy's performance at the 2007 Walker Cup that truly solidified his reputation as a force to be reckoned with in amateur golf. Representing Great Britain and Ireland, McIlroy delivered a standout

The Drive of Rory McIlroy

performance, winning all four of his matches and playing a pivotal role in his team's victory over the United States. His stellar play and unwavering composure under pressure showcased his ability to perform on the biggest stages, setting the stage for what would be a remarkable professional career.

As McIlroy transitioned to the professional ranks, he carried with him the invaluable experience and confidence gained from his time as an amateur. His successes on the amateur circuit not only served as a testament to his talent but also provided him with the necessary foundation to thrive at the highest level of the sport.

Today, Rory McIlroy stands as one of the most accomplished golfers of his generation, with numerous major championships and accolades to his name. Yet, it is his journey as an amateur golfer, marked by unparalleled successes and defining moments, that truly embodies the essence of his legendary status in the world of golf.

2.3: Decision to Turn Professional

Rory McIlroy's decision to turn professional was not merely a leap of faith but a meticulously calculated career move that would ultimately shape the trajectory of his golfing journey. As one of the most talented amateurs in the game, McIlroy faced the pivotal choice of when to make the transition to the professional ranks, balancing the allure of potential success with the inherent risks and challenges that accompany such a significant step.

McIlroy's journey to professionalism was marked by a series of pivotal moments and considerations. Despite his youth, his exceptional talent and undeniable potential had already garnered widespread attention within the golfing community. As he continued to excel on the amateur circuit, capturing titles and accolades with remarkable consistency, the pressure mounted for him to take the next step in his career.

One of the key factors influencing McIlroy's decision was his desire to compete against the best players in the world on a regular basis. While he had achieved significant success as an amateur, including victories in prestigious tournaments and events, McIlroy recognised that the professional ranks offered a new level of competition and opportunity for growth.

Furthermore, McIlroy's team, including his family, coaches, and advisors, played a crucial role in guiding his decision-making process. Together, they carefully evaluated the pros and cons of turning professional at various stages of his development, taking into account factors such as his skill level, mental readiness, and financial considerations.

Ultimately, the timing of McIlroy's decision to turn professional was influenced by a combination of factors, including his age, experience, and confidence in his abilities. In 2007, at the age of 18, McIlroy made the momentous announcement that he would be foregoing his amateur status to pursue a career in professional golf.

The transition to professionalism was not without its challenges for McIlroy. As he embarked on the journey to establish himself as a force to be reckoned with on the PGA Tour, he faced the pressures of heightened

The Drive of Rory McIlroy

expectations, increased scrutiny, and the need to adapt to the rigours of competing at the highest level of the sport.

However, McIlroy's decision to turn professional ultimately proved to be a masterstroke, setting the stage for a career defined by unparalleled success and achievement. With his unwavering dedication, exceptional talent, and relentless pursuit of excellence, McIlroy quickly rose through the ranks to become one of the most dominant forces in golf, capturing major championships, ascending to the top of the world rankings, and etching his name into the annals of the sport's history.

In hindsight, McIlroy's decision to turn professional represented not only a pivotal moment in his own career but also a testament to his foresight, ambition, and unwavering belief in his ability to compete and succeed at the highest level.

CHAPTER 3: THE JOURNEY TO STARDOM:

A Tale of Talent, Tenacity, and Triumph

Rory McIlroy's journey to stardom is a captivating narrative of raw talent, unwavering determination, and remarkable triumphs against all odds. From his humble beginnings in Northern Ireland to his ascent to the summit of professional golf, McIlroy's path to greatness is characterised by a series of defining moments and extraordinary achievements that have solidified his status as one of the sport's most iconic figures.

McIlroy's love affair with golf began at an early age, nurtured by his supportive family and fueled by his innate passion for the game. Gifted with natural talent and a fierce competitive spirit, he quickly emerged as a

The Drive of Rory McIlroy

standout junior golfer, turning heads with his prodigious skill and precocious ability to excel under pressure.

One of the pivotal moments in McIlroy's journey came in 20072007, when, at the age of 18, he made the bold decision to turn professional. Armed with unwavering self-belief and an insatiable hunger for success, McIlroy embarked on a quest to establish himself as a force to be reckoned with on the global stage.

McIlroy's early years as a professional were marked by flashes of brilliance and glimpses of his immense potential. He wasted no time in making his presence felt, capturing his first professional win at the 2009 Dubai Desert Classic and announcing himself as a rising star in the world of golf.

However, it was McIlroy's breakthrough victory at the 2011 U.S. Open that catapulted him into the stratosphere of superstardom. With a breathtaking display of skill and composure, McIlroy stormed to victory atat the Congressional Country Club, becoming the youngest winner of the U.S. Open since 1923 and cementing his status as one of the game's brightest talents.

The Drive of Rory McIlroy

From that moment onward, McIlroy's star continued to rise as he amassed an impressive array of titles and accolades on both sides of the Atlantic. His electrifying performances, fearless demeanourdemeanour, and unwavering commitment to excellence endeared him to fans around the world, while his rivalry with fellow icons such as Tiger Woods and Jordan Spieth added an extra layer of drama and intrigue to the sport.

Throughout his career, McIlroy has faced his fair share of challenges and setbacks, from injury woes to periods of inconsistency on the course. Yet, through it all, he has remained resolute in his pursuit of greatness, drawing strength from adversity and using it as fuel to propel himself to even greater heights.

Today, Rory McIlroy stands as one of the most accomplished golfers of his generation, with multiple major championships, FedEx Cup titles, and Ryder Cup triumphs to his name. Yet, beyond the trophies and accolades, it is McIlroy's unwavering passion for the game, his relentless work ethic, and his unwavering commitment to excellence that truly define his journey to stardom. In an era defined by fierce competition and fleeting fame, McIlroy's enduring legacy serves as a testament to the power of talent, tenacity, and triumph in the face of adversity.

3.1: Early Professional Career Challenges

Rory McIlroy's early professional career was marked by a series of challenges and obstacles that tested his resilience, character, and resolve. Despite his prodigious talent and immense potential, McIlroy faced a steep learning curve as he navigated the transition from amateur sensation to professional contender on the world stage.

One of the most notable challenges McIlroy encountered early in his professional career was the pressure of heightened expectations. As a highly touted prospect with a string of amateur victories to his name, McIlroy faced immense scrutiny and sky-high expectations from fans, media, and sponsors alike. The weight of these expectations, coupled with the relentless demands of

The Drive of Rory McIlroy

professional golf, placed a significant burden on McIlroy's shoulders and tested his mental fortitude.

Another major challenge for McIlroy was adapting to the rigours of professional competition. Unlike the amateur ranks, where success is often measured in individual tournaments and titles, the professional circuit demands consistency and resilience over the course of an entire season. McIlroy struggled at times to find his footing in this new environment, grappling with the physical and mental demands of competing week in and week out against the world's best players.

In addition to the external pressures and demands of professional golf, McIlroy also faced internal challenges and doubts. Like any young athlete, he grappled with moments of self-doubt and uncertainty, questioning whether he had what it took to succeed at the highest level. However, it was McIlroy's unwavering self-belief and unyielding determination that ultimately enabled him to overcome these challenges and persevere in the face of adversity.

The Drive of Rory McIlroy

One of the most significant setbacks McIlroy faced in his early professional career came in the form of an injury. an injury. In 2015, he suffered a ruptured ankle ligament while playing soccer, forcing him to withdraw from the Open Championship and putting his season in jeopardy. The injury served as a stark reminder of the physical toll that professional golf can take on the body and forced McIlroy to confront his own mortality and vulnerability as an athlete.

Despite these challenges, McIlroy remained steadfast in his commitment to excellence and continued to hone his craft with unwavering determination. He sought guidance from mentors and coaches, fine-tuned his skills through hours of practice and repetition, and embraced the lessons learned from both triumphs and setbacks along the way.

In hindsight, McIlroy's early professional career challenges served as valuable learning experiences that ultimately shaped him into the champion he is today. They taught him resilience in the face of adversity, humility in the midst of success, and the importance of perseverance in the pursuit of greatness.

The Drive of Rory McIlroy

Today, Rory McIlroy stands as one of the most accomplished golfers of his generation, with multiple major championships and accolades to his name. Yet, it is his journey through adversity and his ability to overcome challenges that truly define his early professional career and serve as a testament to his character, determination, and unwavering commitment to excellence.

3.2: Breakthrough Wins and Notable Performances

Rory McIlroy's career has been punctuated by a series of breakthrough wins and notable performances that have solidified his status as one of the most dominant forces in golf. From his early triumphs to his major championship victories and historic achievements, McIlroy's journey to greatness is characterised by moments of brilliance and unparalleled skill on the biggest stages of the sport.

The Drive of Rory McIlroy

One of McIlroy's earliest breakthrough wins came at the age of 19, when he captured his maiden European Tour title at the 2009 Dubai Desert Classic. Displaying a maturity beyond his years and a flair for the dramatic, McIlroy held off a star-studded field to secure a one-stroke victory and announce himself as a rising star in the world of golf.

However, it was McIlroy's victory at the 2011 U.S. Open that truly catapulted him into the spotlight and solidified his reputation as a major championship contender. With a breathtaking display of skill and composure, McIlroy dominated the field at Congressional Country Club, finishing with a record-breaking score of 16-under-par to claim his first major title. At just 22 years old, McIlroy became the youngest U.S. Open champion since Bobby Jones in 1923, cementing his status as one of the game's brightest talents.

McIlroy's success at the 2011 U.S. Open served as a springboard for further triumphs on the world stage. In 2012, he captured his second major championship victory at the PGA Championship, holding off a late charge from a formidable field to claim the Wanamaker Trophy and etch his name into the annals of golfing

The Drive of Rory McIlroy

history. With this victory, McIlroy became the youngest player since Seve Ballesteros to win multiple major championships, further solidifying his status as a generational talent.

In the years that followed, McIlroy continued to showcase his dominance on the PGA Tour and the European Tour, amassing an impressive array of titles and accolades. His performances at prestigious events such as the Masters Tournament, the Open Championship, and the Ryder Cup further cemented his reputation as one of the most formidable competitors in the game, while his unwavering commitment to excellence and his relentless pursuit of greatness endeared him to fans around the world.

One of the most notable performances of McIlroy's career came at the 2014 Open Championship, where he delivered a masterful display of golf to claim the Claret Jug and secure his third major championship victory. Trailing by six shots after the opening round, McIlroy produced a stunning comeback, shooting rounds of 66-66-68 to storm to victory and cement his status as one of the game's elite players.

The Drive of Rory McIlroy

In addition to his individual successes, McIlroy has also enjoyed remarkable achievements on the international stage, representing Europe with distinction in the Ryder Cup and playing a pivotal role in his team's triumphs over the United States. His passion, determination, and unwavering commitment to excellence have made him a beloved figure in the world of golf and a true ambassador for the sport.

Today, Rory McIlroy stands as one of the most accomplished golfers of his generation, with multiple major championships, FedEx Cup titles, and Ryder Cup triumphs to his name. Yet, beyond the trophies and accolades, it is McIlroy's enduring legacy as a pioneer, a competitor, and a champion that truly defines his remarkable career and cements his place in the pantheon of golfing greatness.

3.3: Establishing a Name on the PGA Tour

Rory McIlroy's journey to establishing himself as one of the most dominant forces on the PGA Tour is a testament

The Drive of Rory McIlroy

to his unwavering talent, relentless determination, and insatiable hunger for success. From his early forays onto the American circuit to his ascendance to the summit of professional golf, McIlroy's path to prominence on the PGA Tour is marked by a series of defining moments and remarkable achievements that have solidified his status as one of the sport's true icons.

McIlroy's first breakthrough on the PGA Tour came in 20102010, when he captured his maiden victory at the Wells Fargo Championship. In a performance that showcased his raw talent and fearless demeanourdemeanour, McIlroy surged to a four-stroke victory, holding off a star-studded field to claim his first PGA Tour title. The win served as a harbinger of things to come, as McIlroy embarked on a meteoric rise through the ranks of professional golf.

One of the defining moments in McIlroy's career came in 20122012, when he captured his second major championship victory at the PGA Championship. With a flawless display of precision and power, McIlroy dominated the field at Kiawah Island's Ocean Course, finishing a staggering eight strokes clear of the nearest competitor to claim the Wanamaker Trophy. The victory

The Drive of Rory McIlroy

not only solidified McIlroy's status as a major championship contender but also established him as a force to be reckoned with on the PGA Tour.

In the years that followed, McIlroy continued to assert his dominance on the PGA Tour, amassing an impressive array of victories and accolades. His performances at prestigious events such as the Players Championship, the Arnold Palmer Invitational, and the Tour Championship further cemented his reputation as one of the most formidable competitors in the game, while his unwavering commitment to excellence and his relentless pursuit of greatness endeared him to fans around the world.

One of the most notable achievements of McIlroy's career came in 20192019, when he captured the FedEx Cup title for the second time. With a commanding display of skill and determination, McIlroy outlasted the competition to claim the coveted FedEx Cup trophy and solidify his status as the PGA Tour's premier player. The victory capped off a remarkable season for McIlroy, during which he recorded multiple wins and consistently performed at the highest level.

The Drive of Rory McIlroy

In addition to his individual successes, McIlroy has also played a pivotal role in elevating the profile of the PGA Tour on the global stage. His charisma, sportsmanship, and unwavering commitment to excellence have made him a beloved figure in the world of golf and a true ambassador for the sport, while his rivalry with fellow icons such as Tiger Woods and Jordan Spieth has added an extra layer of drama and intrigue to the PGA Tour.

Today, Rory McIlroy stands as one of the most accomplished golfers of his generation, with multiple major championships, FedEx Cup titles, and Ryder Cup triumphs to his name. Yet, beyond the trophies and accolades, it is McIlroy's enduring legacy as a pioneer, a competitor, and a champion that truly defines his remarkable career and cements his place as one of the greatest players in the history of the PGA Tour.

CHAPTER 4: MAJOR TRIUMPH:

Triumphs on Golf's Grandest Stage

Rory McIlroy's major triumphs stand as the crowning achievements of his illustrious career, defining him as one of the greatest golfers of his generation. From his electrifying breakthrough at the U.S. Open to his historic victories at the Open Championship and PGA Championship, McIlroy's dominance on golf's grandest stages has solidified his legacy as a true champion.

McIlroy's first major victory came at the 2011 U.S. Open, held atat the Congressional Country Club. With a breathtaking display of precision and power, McIlroy showcased his unrivalled talent and unwavering

The Drive of Rory McIlroy

composure to claim his maiden major championship. Finishing with a record-breaking score of 16-under-par, McIlroy became the youngest U.S. Open champion since 1923, announcing himself as a force to be reckoned with on the world stage.

Following his triumph at the U.S. Open, McIlroy continued his major championship success with a stunning victory at the 2012 PGA Championship. Held at Kiawah Island's Ocean Course, McIlroy delivered a masterclass in golfing excellence, surging to an eight-stroke victory to claim his second major title. His dominant performance solidified his status as one of the game's premier players and marked him as a true contender for golf's most prestigious honours.

McIlroy's major triumphs continued in 2014 when he captured the Claret Jug at the Open Championship, held at Royal Liverpool Golf Club. Trailing by six shots after the opening round, McIlroy produced a remarkable comeback, showcasing his resilience and determination to claim victory. With a display of skill and precision under pressure, McIlroy secured his third major championship title and further cemented his legacy as one of the game's all-time greats.

The Drive of Rory McIlroy

In addition to his individual successes, McIlroy has also played a pivotal role in leading Team Europe to victory in the Ryder Cup, further solidifying his status as one of the most accomplished golfers of his generation. His passion, leadership, and unwavering commitment to excellence have made him a beloved figure in the world of golf and a true ambassador for the sport.

Today, Rory McIlroy stands as one of the most decorated golfers in history, with multiple major championships, FedEx Cup titles, and Ryder Cup triumphs to his name. Yet, beyond the trophies and accolades, it is McIlroy's enduring legacy as a pioneer, a competitor, and a champion that truly defines his remarkable career and cements his place as one of the greatest players to ever grace the fairways.

4.1: The Quest for Major Championship

Rory McIlroy's quest for major championships is a compelling narrative of triumphs, trials, and unwavering determination in the pursuit of golfing greatness. From his early aspirations as a young prodigy to his emergence

The Drive of Rory McIlroy

as one of the sport's most dominant figures, McIlroy's journey to major championship success is marked by moments of brilliance, heartbreak, and unyielding resolve.

McIlroy's quest for major championships began at an early age, fueled by his innate talent and burning desire to etch his name into the annals of golfing history. As a young amateur, McIlroy dreamt of competing against the best in the world on golf's grandest stages, envisioning himself hoisting the iconic trophies of the sport's most prestigious events.

One of the defining moments in McIlroy's quest for major championships came at the 2011 U.S. Open, held atat the Congressional Country Club. With a display of golfing virtuosity that captivated the world, McIlroy stormed to victory, finishing with a record-breaking score of 16-under-par to claim his maiden major title. The win not only solidified McIlroy's status as a major championship contender but also instilled in him a hunger for further success on golf's grandest stages.

The Drive of Rory McIlroy

Despite his early triumph at the U.S. Open, McIlroy's quest for major championships would prove to be a journey fraught with challenges and setbacks. From heartbreaking losses inin the playoffs to battles with injury and inconsistency, McIlroy faced his fair share of adversity on the road to major glory. Yet, through it all, he remained steadfast in his belief in his ability to overcome obstacles and emerge stronger on the other side.

McIlroy's perseverance and resilience were on full display at the 2014 Open Championship, held atat the Royal Liverpool Golf Club. Trailing by six shots after the opening round, McIlroy staged a remarkable comeback, showcasing his mental fortitude and competitive spirit to claim victory and secure his third major championship title. The win served as a testament to McIlroy's unwavering resolve and his ability to rise to the occasion when it mattered most.

In the years that followed, McIlroy continued his quest for major championships with unwavering determination, adding to his trophy cabinet with victories at the PGA Championship and the Players Championship, among others. While the road to major glory has been fraught with challenges and obstacles, McIlroy's unwavering commitment to excellence and his relentless pursuit of greatness have positioned him as one of the most formidable contenders in the history of the sport.

Rory McIlroy stands as one of the most accomplished golfers of his generation, with multiple major championships and accolades to his name. Yet, beyond the trophies and accolades, it is McIlroy's enduring legacy as a pioneer, a competitor, and a champion that truly defines his remarkable quest for major championships and cements his place as one of the greatest players to ever grace the fairways.

4.2: The 2011 U.S. Open Victory

Rory McIlroy's victory at the 2011 U.S. Open stands as one of the defining moments of his career, a breathtaking display of golfing brilliance that announced his arrival as one of the sport's most formidable talents. From his record-breaking performance to the sheer dominance he exhibited over the course of four unforgettable days,

The Drive of Rory McIlroy

McIlroy's triumph at Congressional Country Club is etched into the annals of golfing history as a milestone achievement.

The stage was set for McIlroy's historic victory at the U.S. Open, held at the venerable Congressional Country Club in Bethesda, Maryland. From the outset, McIlroy's sublime ball-striking and impeccable course management captured the attention of fans and competitors alike, as he surged to the top of the leaderboard with a flawless opening round of 65.

As the tournament progressed, McIlroy continued to dazzle with his precision and poise, extending his lead with each passing round. His mastery of the demanding layout at Congressional was on full display as he navigated treacherous hazards and daunting greens with apparent ease, showcasing a level of skill and maturity beyond his years.

By the time the final round arrived, McIlroy had firmly established himself as the player to beat, holding a commanding lead over the field. Despite the pressure and expectation that comecome with leading a major

The Drive of Rory McIlroy

championship, McIlroy remained composed and focused, determined to seize his moment and etch his name into the annals of golfing history.

In a performance for the ages, McIlroy delivered a masterclass in golfing excellence, closing out the tournament with a record-breaking score of 16-under-par to claim his maiden major championship title. His final-round score of 69 was a testament to his mental fortitude and unwavering resolve, as he maintained his composure under the intense scrutiny of the golfing world and emerged victorious in spectacular fashion.

McIlroy's victory at the 2011 U.S. Open was not merely a triumph on the golf course but a transcendent moment that captured the imagination of fans around the world. His grace, humility, and sportsmanship in victory endeared him to fans and fellow competitors alike, while his sheer dominance over the field solidified his status as a major championship contender for years to come.

In the years since his historic victory at Congressional, McIlroy has gone on to achieve further success on golf's grandest stages, adding multiple major championship titles to his illustrious resume. Yet, it is his triumph at the 2011 U.S. Open that remains etched in the collective memory of golf fans everywhere, a shining example of excellence and achievement in the face of adversity.

4.3: Masters, Open Championships, and PGA Championship Successes

Rory McIlroy's success in the Masters, Open Championships, and PGA Championship has solidified his status as one of the greatest golfers of his generation. From his remarkable breakthrough at the U.S. Open to his triumphs at golf's most prestigious events, McIlroy's major championship victories represent the pinnacle of his illustrious career and a testament to his unwavering talent, determination, and tenacity.

McIlroy's quest for major championship success began in earnest at the 2011 U.S. Open, where he captured his maiden major title in record-breaking fashion. From there, McIlroy continued his ascent to greatness with victories at the Open Championship and the PGA Championship, etching his name into the annals of golfing history and solidifying his legacy as one of the sport's true icons.

The Drive of Rory McIlroy

One of McIlroy's most memorable major triumphs came at the 2014 Open Championship, held atat the Royal Liverpool Golf Club. Trailing by six shots after the opening round, McIlroy staged a remarkable comeback, showcasing his resilience and determination to claim victory and secure his third major championship title. His performance at Royal Liverpool was a testament to his ability to rise to the occasion when it mattered most, solidifying his status as one of the game's premier players.

In addition to his victory at the Open Championship, McIlroy has also enjoyed success at the PGA Championship, one of golf's most prestigious events. His triumph at the 2012 PGA Championship, held at Kiawah Island's Ocean Course, was a masterclass in golfing excellence, as McIlroy surged to an eight-stroke victory to claim his second major championship title. His dominant performance at Kiawah Island further cemented his status as one of the sport's all-time greats and set the stage for further success on golf's grandest stages.

The Drive of Rory McIlroy

McIlroy's success in the Masters, golf's most revered tournament, has been a focal point of his career and a source of both triumph and heartbreak. While he has yet to claim the coveted green jacket, McIlroy has been a perennial contender at Augusta National, with multiple top-10 finishes to his name. His quest for Masters glory remains an ongoing pursuit, as he continues to chase his dream of completing the career Grand Slam and etching his name into the annals of golfing immortality.

In the years since his historic breakthrough at the U.S. Open, McIlroy has continued to assert his dominance on golf's grandest stages, adding to his trophy cabinet with victories at the Players Championship, the FedEx Cup, and numerous other prestigious events. Yet, it is his success in the Masters, Open Championships, and PGA Championship that stand as the crowning achievements of his illustrious career and a testament to his enduring legacy as one of the greatest golfers of all time.

The Drive of Rory McIlroy

CHAPTER 5: THE MENTAL GAME

The Driving Force Behind a Golfing Legend

Rory McIlroy's mental game is often cited as one of the driving forces behind his success on the golf course. From his unwavering focus and resilience to his ability to perform under pressure, McIlroy's mental fortitude has set him apart as one of the most formidable competitors in the sport. Delving into the intricacies of McIlroy's mental approach reveals a mindset characterized by discipline, determination, and an unwavering belief in his ability to succeed.

One of the hallmarks of McIlroy's mental game is his ability to maintain focus and composure under the most challenging circumstances. Whether facing a daunting tee shot on the final hole of a major championship or navigating a treacherous stretch of holes during a crucial round, McIlroy's calm demeanour and laser-like focus enable him to block out distractions and stay fully present in the moment. This ability to maintain mental clarity and stay in the zone has been instrumental in

The Drive of Rory McIlroy

McIlroy's success on the golf course, allowing him to perform at his best when it matters most.

In addition to his ability to stay focused under pressure, McIlroy's mental game is characterised by a relentless pursuit of excellence and a refusal to settle for anything less than his best. Known for his tireless work ethic and commitment to improvement, McIlroy approaches each round with a hunger for success and a determination to push the boundaries of his own potential. Whether fine-tuning his swing on the practice range or meticulously studying course conditions and strategy, McIlroy leaves no stone unturned in his quest for perfection.

Another key aspect of McIlroy's mental game is his resilience in the face of adversity. Like any athlete, McIlroy has faced his fair share of setbacks and challenges throughout his career, from injury woes to periods of poor form. Yet, it is his ability to bounce back from adversity with renewed determination and resolve that truly sets him apart as a champion. Rather than dwelling on past failures or setbacks, McIlroy uses them as fuel to drive him forward, learning from his mistakes and emerging stronger and more resilient as a result.

Perhaps most importantly, McIlroy's mental game is underpinned by a deep-seated belief in his ability to succeed. From a young age, McIlroy has possessed an unshakeable confidence in his own talents and a firm belief that he has what it takes to compete and win at the highest level. This self-belief has been a constant source of strength and motivation for McIlroy throughout his career, empowering him to push the boundaries of his own potential and achieve greatness on the golf course.

Rory McIlroy's mental game is a testament to the power of discipline, determination, and self-belief in the pursuit of excellence. From his unwavering focus and resilience to his relentless pursuit of perfection, McIlroy's mental approach sets him apart as one of the greatest golfers of his generation and a true legend of the sport.

5.1: Mental Toughness and Resilience

Rory McIlroy's mental toughness and resilience are the bedrock of his success on the golf course, serving as the guiding forces that have propelled him through triumphs

The Drive of Rory McIlroy

and setbacks alike. From his ability to bounce back from adversity to his unwavering focus under pressure, McIlroy's mental fortitude has been a defining characteristic of his illustrious career, shaping him into one of the most formidable competitors in the sport.

At the core of McIlroy's mental toughness is his remarkable ability to maintain perspective and resilience in the face of adversity. Throughout his career, McIlroy has faced his fair share of challenges, from injury setbacks to periods of poor form and disappointing performances. Yet, rather than succumbing to doubt or despair, McIlroy has consistently demonstrated an uncanny ability to bounce back from setbacks with renewed determination and resolve. This resilience in the face of adversity has been instrumental in McIlroy's ability to weather the storms of professional golf and emerge stronger and more resilient on the other side.

In addition to his resilience in the face of adversity, McIlroy's mental toughness is characterised by his unwavering focus and composure under pressure. Whether contending for a major championship or facing a crucial shot with the tournament on the line, McIlroy has a remarkable ability to block out distractions and stay fully present in the moment. This ability to maintain mental clarity and stay in the zone under the most pressure-packed circumstances has been a key factor in McIlroy's ability to perform at his best when it matters most, consistently delivering clutch performances on the game's grandest stages.

Furthermore, McIlroy's mental toughness is underpinned by his unwavering self-belief and confidence in his abilities. From a young age, McIlroy has possessed an unshakeable belief in his own talents and a firm conviction that he has what it takes to compete and win at the highest level. This self-belief has been a constant source of strength and motivation for McIlroy throughout his career, empowering him to push the boundaries of his own potential and achieve greatness on the golf course.

Another key aspect of McIlroy's mental toughness is his ability to learn and grow from his experiences, both positive and negative. Whether celebrating a victory or analysing a defeat, McIlroy approaches each outcome as an opportunity for growth and improvement, constantly striving to refine his skills and sharpen his mental game. This growth mindset has been instrumental in McIlroy's ability to evolve as a player and continue to raise the bar for excellence in the sport.

Rory McIlroy's mental toughness and resilience are the cornerstones of his success on the golf course, enabling him to navigate the highs and lows of professional golf with grace, poise, and unwavering determination. From his ability to bounce back from setbacks to his unwavering focus under pressure, McIlroy's mental fortitude sets him apart as one of the greatest competitors in the history of the sport, a true testament to the power of the mind in the pursuit of excellence.

5.2:Overcoming Setbacks and Challenges

Rory McIlroy's journey to the pinnacle of professional golf has been marked by a series of setbacks and challenges, each of which he has met with unwavering resilience and determination. From injury woes to periods of poor form and disappointing performances, McIlroy's ability to overcome adversity has been a

The Drive of Rory McIlroy

defining characteristic of his illustrious career, shaping him into one of the sport's most formidable competitors.

One of the most notable setbacks McIlroy faced early in his career came in 2011, when he endured a highly publicised collapse at the Masters Tournament. Holding a commanding lead heading into the final round, McIlroy struggled to find his rhythm and ultimately faltered down the stretch, finishing tied for 15th place. While the defeat was undoubtedly painful, McIlroy refused to let it define him, using it as motivation to redouble his efforts and sharpen his mental game for future challenges.

Another significant setback for McIlroy came in 2015 when he suffered a ruptured ankle ligament while playing soccer, forcing him to withdraw from the Open Championship and putting his season in jeopardy. The injury served as a stark reminder of the physical toll that professional golf can take on the body and forced McIlroy to confront his own mortality and vulnerability as an athlete. Yet, rather than allowing the setback to derail his career, McIlroy embraced the challenge head-on, undergoing rigorous rehabilitation and rededicating himself to his craft with renewed vigour.

The Drive of Rory McIlroy

In addition to these high-profile setbacks, McIlroy has also faced periods of poor form and disappointing performances throughout his career. From struggles with his swing to bouts of inconsistency on the course, McIlroy has experienced his fair share of ups and downs on the journey to greatness. Yet, through it all, he has remained steadfast in his belief in his own abilities and his commitment to the pursuit of excellence, refusing to let setbacks define him or deter him from his ultimate goals.

One of the most remarkable aspects of McIlroy's ability to overcome setbacks is his unwavering resilience and determination in the face of adversity. Rather than dwelling on past failures or succumbing to doubt and despair, McIlroy uses setbacks as fuel to drive him forward, learning from his mistakes and emerging stronger and more resilient as a result. His ability to bounce back from setbacks with renewed determination and resolve is a testament to his mental toughness and his unwavering belief in his ability to succeed.

Rory McIlroy's ability to overcome setbacks and challenges throughout his career is a testament to his resilience, determination, and unwavering belief in his ability to succeed. From high-profile collapses to injury woes and periods of poor form, McIlroy has faced his fair share of adversity on the journey to greatness. Yet, through it all, he has remained steadfast in his commitment to the pursuit of excellence, using setbacks as opportunities for growth and learning and emerging stronger and more resilient on the other side.

5.3:Mindset and Approach to Pressure Situations

Rory McIlroy's mindset and approach to pressure situations have long been admired and studied by golf enthusiasts and sports psychologists alike. From his unwavering focus and calm demeanor under the spotlight to his ability to thrive in high-pressure moments, McIlroy's mental fortitude is a key factor in his success on the golf course.

The Drive of Rory McIlroy

At the heart of McIlroy's approach to pressure situations is his ability to stay present and focused in the moment. Whether contending for a major championship or facing a crucial shot with the tournament on the line, McIlroy has an uncanny ability to block out distractions and stay fully engaged in the task at hand. This mental clarity allows him to maintain a heightened sense of awareness and make sound decisions under pressure, giving him a competitive edge when it matters most.

In addition to his ability to stay present, McIlroy's mindset in pressure situations is characterised by his embrace of the challenge and his confidence in his own abilities. Rather than viewing pressure as a hindrance or a source of anxiety, McIlroy sees it as an opportunity to showcase his skills and rise to the occasion. His unwavering self-belief and confidence in his ability to perform under pressure enable him to approach each challenge with a sense of calm and poise, allowing him to deliver his best when it matters most.

Another key aspect of McIlroy's mindset in pressure situations is his ability to embrace the moment and trust in his preparation. Through meticulous practice and preparation, McIlroy ensures that he is fully equipped to

The Drive of Rory McIlroy

handle the demands of competition, both physically and mentally. This preparation instills in him a sense of confidence and assurance, knowing that he has done everything in his power to be ready for whatever challenges lie ahead.

Furthermore, McIlroy's mindset in stressfulstressful situations is underpinned by his ability to maintain perspective and focus on the process rather than the outcome. Rather than allowing himself to become overwhelmed by the magnitude of the moment, McIlroy breaks down the challenge into manageable steps and focuses on executing each shot to the best of his ability. This approach helps him to stay grounded and composed under pressure, enabling him to perform at his best when it matters most.

Rory McIlroy's mindset and approach to pressure situations are characterized by a combination of focus, confidence, and preparation. His ability to stay present, embrace the challenge, and trust in his abilities has enabled him to thrive in high-pressure moments and emerge as one of the most formidable competitors in the history of the sport. Whether contending for major championships or facing adversity on the course, McIlroy's mental mastery is a key factor in his success and a testament to his unwavering determination and resilience.

CHAPTER 6: TECHNIQUES AND TRAINING

Rory McIlroy, one of golf's most prominent figures, possesses a technique and training regimen that epitomise excellence in the sport. His prowess on the golf course is a testament to his meticulous approach to both physical and mental preparation.

Technique:

1. Swing mechanics: McIlroy's swing is characterised by its fluidity and power. He generates tremendous clubhead speed through a combination of proper sequencing, efficient weight transfer, and a full rotation of the hips and shoulders.

2. Grip: His grip is strong, promoting a controlled release through impact while minimising the risk of hooks or slices.

3. Stance and posture: McIlroy maintains a balanced stance with slightly bent knees,

allowing for stability throughout the swing. His posture is athletic, ensuring optimal alignment and weight distribution.

4. Timing and Rhythm: His swing's timing and rhythm are impeccable, resulting in consistent ball-striking and distance control.

5. Short Game: McIlroy's short game is equally impressive, characterised by deft touch and creativity around the greens. His ability to execute delicate pitches and precise chip shots sets him apart from his peers.

Training:

1. Physical Conditioning: McIlroy dedicates significant time to physical training, focusing on strength, flexibility, and cardiovascular fitness. His workouts include weightlifting, plyometrics, and exercises targeting core stability.

2. Golf-Specific Drills: He incorporates drills designed to hone specific aspects of his game, such as tempo drills to refine his swing rhythm and short game drills to improve his feel around the greens.

3. Technical Analysis: McIlroy works closely with his coaches and utilises cutting-edge technology, such as launch monitors and swing analysis software, to dissect his swing mechanics and identify areas for improvement.

4. Mental Preparation: Mental toughness is paramount in golf, and McIlroy places great emphasis on mental preparation. He practices visualisation techniques to envision successful shots and employs mindfulness exercises to stay focused and composed under pressure.

5. Competition Simulation: To simulate tournament conditions, McIlroy often engages in practice rounds with fellow professionals or competes in

friendly matches with high stakes on the line. This helps him acclimatise to the pressure of competitive golf and fine-tune his decision-making skills.

6. Rest and Recovery: Recognising the importance of rest and recovery in optimising performance, McIlroy prioritise adequate sleep, proper nutrition, and recovery modalities such as massage and stretching to ensure his body is primed for peak performance.

Rory McIlroy's technique and training regimen serve as a blueprint for aspiring golfers looking to reach the pinnacle of the sport. Through relentless dedication, attention to detail, and a holistic approach to physical and mental preparation, McIlroy continues to cement his legacy as one of golf's all-time greats.

6.1: The Evolution of Rory McIlroy's Swing

The Drive of Rory McIlroy

Rory McIlroy's swing has undergone a fascinating evolution throughout his career, marked by refinement, experimentation, and adaptation to changing circumstances. Let's delve into the key stages of this evolution:

Early Years:

1. Natural Talent: From a young age, McIlroy displayed prodigious talent and a technically sound swing. His fluid, athletic motion caught the attention of coaches and observers, foreshadowing future success.

2. Amateur Development: As a junior and amateur golfer, McIlroy's swing continued to evolve under the guidance of coaches who helped him fine-tune his mechanics and develop a reliable ball flight.

Breakthrough Years:

The Drive of Rory McIlroy

1. Professional Debut: McIlroy burst onto the professional scene with a swing characterized by raw power and aggressive tempo. His youthful exuberance and fearlessness endeared him to fans, while his ability to generate prodigious distance off the tee garnered widespread acclaim.

2. Major Victories: With each major championship victory, McIlroy's swing underwent subtle adjustments aimed at improving consistency and shot-making versatility. His win at the 2011 U.S. Open showcased his ability to dominate a major championship with a combination of precision iron play and long, towering drives.

Mid-Career Adjustments:

1. Equipment Changes: McIlroy's transition to new equipment sponsors prompted adjustments to his swing to optimise performance with his new gear. These adjustments often involved fine-tuning launch angles, spin rates, and ball

flight characteristics to maximise distance and accuracy.

2. Technical Tweaks: McIlroy continued to refine his swing mechanics under the guidance of renowned coaches, incorporating elements from the latest advances in biomechanics and swing analysis technology. These tweaks focused on maintaining balance, improving clubface control, and optimising swing sequencing for maximum efficiency.

Recent Developments:

1. Age and Experience: As McIlroy has matured as a golfer, his swing has evolved to reflect a deeper understanding of his own strengths and weaknesses. He has learned to temper his aggression when necessary, opting for controlled aggression and strategic course management in lieu of reckless abandon.

The Drive of Rory McIlroy

2. Short Game Emphasis: In recent years, McIlroy has placed increased emphasis on his short game, recognising its importance in maintaining consistency and minimising scoring errors. His improved proficiency around the greens has complemented his formidable ball-striking prowess, making him a more well-rounded player.

Rory McIlroy's swing evolution is a testament to his commitment to continuous improvement and adaptation in pursuit of excellence. From the raw talent of his early years to the refined precision of his current game, McIlroy's swing embodies the culmination of years of dedication, hard work, and relentless pursuit of perfection. As he continues to compete at the highest levels of professional golf, McIlroy's swing will undoubtedly continue to evolve, ensuring his place among the sport's elite for years to come.

6.2: Training Regimens and Fitness Routines

Rory McIlroy, one of golf's elite players, maintains a rigorous training regimen and fitness routine to stay at the top of his game. His dedication to physical fitness has become a hallmark of his career, allowing him to generate powerful swings, maintain endurance during tournaments, and prevent injuries. Here's a detailed look at Rory McIlroy's training regimens and fitness routines:

1. Strength Training:

McIlroy incorporates strength training to build muscle mass and power. His workouts often focus on compound movements such as squats, deadlifts, and bench presses, which engage multiple muscle groups simultaneously.

He also incorporates exercises specifically targeting golf-related muscles, such as rotational core exercises, to improve his swing mechanics and generate more clubhead speed.

2. Cardiovascular Conditioning:

Cardiovascular fitness is crucial for McIlroy's endurance on the golf course, especially during multi-day tournaments. He includes activities like running, cycling, and rowing in his routine to improve his cardiovascular health and stamina.

High-intensity interval training (HIIT) may also be a part of his cardio regimen, allowing him to push his limits and improve his recovery between rounds.

3. Flexibility and Mobility:

McIlroy understands the importance of flexibility and mobility for a fluid golf swing and injury prevention. He incorporates stretching exercises and yoga into his routine to improve joint range of motion and maintain muscle suppleness.

Yoga also helps him develop core strength, balance, and mental focus, all of which are essential for consistent performance on the golf course.

4. Nutrition:

A well-balanced diet is critical for McIlroy's overall health and performance. He focuses on consuming lean proteins, complex carbohydrates, healthy fats, and plenty of fruits and vegetables to fuel his body for intense training sessions and tournaments.

Proper hydration is also a priority, and he ensures he drinks enough water throughout the day to stay hydrated, especially in hot weather conditions on the golf course.

5. Recovery:

Adequate rest and recovery are essential parts of McIlroy's training regimen to prevent burnout and injuries. He prioritises quality sleep to allow his body to repair and regenerate after intense workouts and rounds of golf.

McIlroy may also utilise recovery modalities such as massage therapy, foam rolling, and ice baths to alleviate muscle soreness and enhance recovery between training sessions and tournaments.

6. Mental Training:

McIlroy recognises the significance of mental toughness and focus in golf. He may engage in mindfulness practices, visualisation techniques, and mental rehearsal to sharpen his concentration and confidence on the course.

Working with sports psychologists or mental coaches may also be part of his routine to develop strategies for managing pressure and maintaining a positive mindset during competition.

Rory McIlroy's training regimens and fitness routines encompass a comprehensive approach to physical and mental preparation for elite-level golf. By prioritising strength, cardiovascular fitness, flexibility, nutrition, recovery, and mental training, McIlroy maximise his potential and consistently performs at the highest level on the golf course.

6.3: Collaborations with Coaches and Experts

Rory McIlroy's collaborations with coaches and experts have played a significant role in shaping his career and maintaining his status as one of golf's elite players. Throughout his journey, McIlroy has sought guidance from various professionals to refine his skills, improve his performance, and stay ahead of the competition. Here's a detailed look at Rory McIlroy's collaborations with coaches and experts:

1. Swing Coaches:

McIlroy has worked with several renowned swing coaches throughout his career, each contributing to the evolution of his swing mechanics and technique.

Notably, he partnered with Michael Bannon, his childhood coach, who played a pivotal role in shaping McIlroy's swing fundamentals and developing his game from a young age.

Additionally, McIlroy has collaborated with esteemed coaches such as Pete Cowen and Dave Stockton, seeking their expertise to fine-tune specific aspects of his swing and short game.

2. Fitness Trainers:

McIlroy's dedication to physical fitness is evident in his collaborations with fitness trainers, who help him maintain peak performance and prevent injuries.

The Drive of Rory McIlroy

He has worked with fitness experts to design personalised training regimens tailored to his golf-specific needs, focusing on strength, flexibility, cardiovascular conditioning, and injury prevention.

These trainers play a crucial role in optimising McIlroy's physical capabilities, enabling him to generate power, endurance, and agility on the golf course.

3. Sports psychologists psychologists psychologists and mentalmental health coacheshealth coaches:

McIlroy recognisesrecognises the importance of mental fortitude and resilience in golf, leading him to collaborate with sports psychologists and mental coaches.

These professionals help McIlroy develop mental strategies to manage pressure, stay focused, and maintain confidence during competition.

Through techniques such as visualisation, mindfulness, and goal-setting, McIlroy strengthens his mental game, enhancing his ability toperform well perform well under stress and adversity.

4. Nutritionists and dietitiansdietitians:

As part of his commitment to peak performance, McIlroy works closely with nutritionists and dietitians to optimise his dietary intake and fuel his body for training and competition.

These experts design customised nutrition plans tailored to McIlroy's energy requirements, ensuring he consumes the right balance of macronutrients and micronutrients to support his physical demands and recovery.

By prioritising proper nutrition and hydration, McIlroy maintains optimal health, energy levels, and performance on the golf course.

5. Biomechanics Specialists:

McIlroy leverages the expertise of biomechanics specialists to analyse his swing mechanics and movement patterns in intricate detail.

Through advanced technologies such as 3D motion analysis and launch monitors, these specialists provide valuable insights into optimising McIlroy's biomechanical efficiency and maximising his swing power and accuracy.

The Drive of Rory McIlroy

By integrating biomechanical feedback into his training and practice routines, McIlroy refines his technique and achieves greater consistency and precision in his ball-striking.

Rory McIlroy's collaborations with coaches and experts span various domains, including swing mechanics, fitness, mental conditioning, nutrition, and biomechanics. By surrounding himself with a team of knowledgeable professionals, McIlroy enhances every aspect of his game, ensuring he remains a dominant force in the world of golf.

CHAPTER 7: OFF THE COURSE

Rory McIlroy is not just a golfing sensation on the course; he's also a fascinating individual off it. Off the course, McIlroy is known for his philanthropy, business ventures, and personal interests.

Philanthropy:

Rory McIlroy is deeply committed to giving back to the community. He established thethe Rory Foundation in 2013, aiming to support children's charities around the world. Through various events and initiatives, the foundation focuses on health, education, and community support for children in need. McIlroy's charitable efforts extend globally, including projects in Ireland, the UK, the United States, and beyond.

Business Ventures:

Beyond golf, McIlroy has ventured into business with strategic investments and partnerships. He's involved in various projects, including endorsements, brand ambassadorships, and entrepreneurial pursuits. Notably, he has endorsement deals with major brands like Nike

The Drive of Rory McIlroy

and TaylorMade, showcasing his influence both on and off the course. Additionally, McIlroy has shown interest in technology startups and real estate investments, diversifying his portfolio beyond the world of golf.

Personal Interests:

Outside of golf and business, McIlroy has diverse interests that reflect his personality. He's an avid sports fan, particularly passionate about soccer and tennis. McIlroy's love for sports extends to his personal life, where he enjoys playing other sports recreationally. Moreover, he's known for his love of cars and occasionally indulges in his passion for fast automobiles. McIlroy's downtime often includes spending time with family and friends, enjoying the simple pleasures of life away from the spotlight.

Family Life:

Family plays a significant role in McIlroy's life. He's married to Erica Stoll, whom he met through his involvement in golf tournaments. Their relationship is a testament to McIlroy's personal life beyond the fairways. The couple often shares glimpses of their liveslives together on social media, portraying a balance between McIlroy's public persona and his private family life.

Rory McIlroy's life off the course is as dynamic as his performance on it. Through philanthropy, business ventures, personal interests, and family life, McIlroy demonstrates a multifaceted personality beyond his golfing prowess. His commitment to making a difference, pursuing diverse interests, and maintaining a balanced personal life showcases the depth of his character beyond the boundaries of golf.

7.1: Personal Life and Interests

Rory McIlroy, the Northern Irish professional golfer, is not only renowned for his remarkable skills on the golf course but also for his intriguing personal life and diverse interests.

Born on May 4, 1989, in Hollywood, County Down, Northern Ireland, Rory McIlroy showed a keen interest in golf from a very young age. His parents, Gerry and

The Drive of Rory McIlroy

Rosie, played a significant role in nurturing his passion for the sport. McIlroy's childhood was filled with rounds of golf at Holywood Golf Club, where he honed his skills and developed his love for the game.

Outside of golf, McIlroy is a multifaceted individual with a variety of interests. He is an avid sports fan, particularly of soccer, and supports both Manchester United and Ulster Rugby. Additionally, he has shown an interest in tennis and has been spotted attending major tournaments such as Wimbledon.

In terms of personal life, McIlroy has been romantically linked with various high-profile figures. He famously dated tennis star Caroline Wozniacki, with whom he was engaged for a brief period before their split in 2014. In 2017, McIlroy married Erica Stoll, a former PGA of America employee, in a lavish ceremony in County Mayo, Ireland. The couple has since welcomed their first child, a daughter named Poppy Kennedy McIlroy, born in August 2020.

Away from the limelight, McIlroy is actively involved in charitable endeavours. He established the Rory

The Drive of Rory McIlroy

Foundation in 2013, which aims to support children's charities around the world. Through his foundation, McIlroy has contributed to various causes, including children's healthcare, education, and community development programmesprogrammes.

Despite his busy schedule, McIlroy also makes time for relaxation and leisure activities. He enjoys travelling to exotic destinations, often sharing glimpses of his adventures on social media. Additionally, he is a self-professed food enthusiast and enjoys exploring different cuisines, both at home and abroad.

Rory McIlroy's personal life reflects a balance between his passion for golf, diverse interests, and commitment to making a positive impact through charitable endeavours. He continues to captivate audiences both on and off the golf course with his talent, charisma, and genuine love for life.

The Drive of Rory McIlroy

7.2:Charitable Endeavours and Giving Back

Rory McIlroy's philanthropic efforts and commitment to giving back have left an indelible mark on communities worldwide. Through his foundation, aptly named the Rory Foundation, McIlroy has embarked on a mission to make a positive impact on the lives of children in need.

Established in 2013, the Rory Foundation focuses on supporting children's charities around the globe. McIlroy, fueled by his own humble beginnings and a desire to give back, has channelled his success and platform as a professional golfer to address various social issues affecting children, including health, education, and community development.

One of the primary initiatives of the Rory Foundation is to provide access to quality healthcare for children facing illness and medical challenges. McIlroy has collaborated with hospitals and healthcare organisations to fund programmesprogrammes and facilities that cater to the specific needs of young patients. These initiatives aim to alleviate the burden on families and ensure that

The Drive of Rory McIlroy

children receive the care and support they require during difficult times.

Education is another cornerstone of the Rory Foundation's efforts. McIlroy believes in the transformative power of education and its ability to unlock opportunities for children from underserved communities. Through scholarships, school infrastructure projects, and educational programmesprogrammes, the foundation endeavours to empower children with the tools they need to succeed academically and pursue their dreams.

Furthermore, the Rory Foundation is actively involved in supporting community development projects that enhance the well-being and prospects of children. Whether it's investing in sports facilities, youth centres, or community outreach programmesprogrammes, McIlroy is dedicated to creating safe and nurturing environments where children can thrive and reach their full potential.

In addition to his foundation's initiatives, McIlroy frequently lends his time, resources, and voice to various charitable causes and fundraising events. He has participated in charity golf tournaments, auctions, and awareness campaigns aimed at raising funds and awareness for issues affecting children.

Beyond financial contributions, McIlroy's hands-on approach to philanthropy has made a tangible difference in the lives of countless children. Whether visiting hospitals, interacting with young patients, or engaging with communities firsthand, McIlroy's genuine compassion and commitment to making a difference have earned him admiration and respect globally.

Rory McIlroy's charitable endeavours exemplify his belief in the power of giving back and his dedication to creating a brighter future for the next generation. By leveraging his platform and resources, McIlroy continues to inspire positive change and leave a lasting legacy of compassion, generosity, and impact.

7.3: Balancing Fame and Privacy

The Drive of Rory McIlroy

Rory McIlroy, a golfing prodigy from Northern Ireland, has garnered worldwide fame and adoration for his exceptional talent on the golf course. However, with fame comes scrutiny, and McIlroy has found himself navigating the delicate balance between enjoying the perks of stardom and safeguarding his privacy.

The Early Years:

McIlroy's rise to fame began at a young age, when he showed promise as a golfer. By his teenage years, he was already making headlines in the golfing world. His natural talent and affable personality endeared him to fans, leading to rapid recognition and sponsorship deals.

The Upside of Fame:

As McIlroy's career flourished, so did his fame. He became a household name, attracting legions of fans and lucrative endorsement deals. His success on the golf course elevated him to the upper echelons of the sport, earning him accolades, titles, and considerable wealth. With fame came opportunities to travel the world, meet influential figures, and enjoy a lifestyle that many could only dream of.

The Drive of Rory McIlroy

The Downside of Fame:

However, with fame came a loss of privacy. McIlroy found himself constantly under the spotlight, with his every move scrutinised by the media and the public alike. Intrusive paparazzi, invasive reporters, and relentless speculation about his personal life became a constant presence. McIlroy struggled to maintain a sense of normalcy amidst the chaos, craving moments of solitude and privacy that seemed increasingly elusive.

Striking a Balance:

Despite the challenges, McIlroy has been proactive in setting boundaries to protect his privacy. He carefully selects which aspects of his life to share with the public, keeping his personal affairs guarded. McIlroy has also prioritised spending quality time with his family and loved ones, cherishing moments away from the limelight.

Moreover, McIlroy has used his platform to advocate for causes close to his heart, leveraging his fame for positive change. Whether through charitable

The Drive of Rory McIlroy

endeavoursendeavours or speaking out on social issues, McIlroy has demonstrated a commitment to making a difference beyond the golf course.

Rory McIlroy's journey serves as a testament to the complexities of fame and privacy in the modern age. While fame has afforded him numerous opportunities and rewards, it has also necessitated careful navigation of public scrutiny and intrusion into his personal life. Through it all, McIlroy remains steadfast in his commitment to balancing the demands of fame with the preservation of his privacy, carving out a path that allows him to thrive both on and off the golf course.

CHAPTER 8: RIVALRIES AND RELATIONSHIPS :

Forging Rivalries and Nurturing Relationships in Golf

Rory McIlroy's journey in the world of golf has been marked by intense rivalries and meaningful relationships, both on and off the course. From his early days as a rising star to his current status as one of the game's elite players, McIlroy's interactions with fellow golfers and his personal connections have played a significant role in shaping his career.

Rivalries on the Course:

Throughout his career, McIlroy has engaged in compelling rivalries with some of the game's greatest players. From his battles with Tiger Woods to his duels with Jordan Spieth and Brooks Koepka, McIlroy has consistently found himself in the midst of intense competition on the fairways and greens.

The Drive of Rory McIlroy

These rivalries have fueled McIlroy's competitive fire, pushing him to elevate his game and strive for excellence. While there is undoubtedly a sense of rivalry on the course, McIlroy has often expressed respect and admiration for his competitors, recognising the role they play in driving him to be his best.

Off-course-course Relationships:

Beyond the competitive arena, McIlroy has cultivated meaningful relationships with his peers, mentors, and fellow professionals. From forging friendships with other golfers to seeking guidance from veteran players, McIlroy has embraced the camaraderie and support network within the golfing community.

McIlroy's relationships extend beyond the world of golf as well. He has a close-knit circle of family and friends who provide unwavering support and encouragement throughout his career. McIlroy's wife, Erica Stoll, whom he married in 2017, has been a constant source of love and stability in his life, accompanying him on tour and celebrating his successes.

The Drive of Rory McIlroy

Navigating Rivalries and Relationships:

While rivalries and relationships are inherent aspects of professional sports, McIlroy has managed to strike a delicate balance between competitiveness and camaraderie. On the course, he approaches his rivals with a mix of determination and respect, recognisingrecognising that their battles ultimately contribute to the greatness of the sport.

Off the course, McIlroy cherishes the relationships he has built, drawing strength and inspiration from the support of his loved ones and peers. He remains grounded in his values and appreciative of the opportunities and friendships that golf has afforded him throughout his career.

Rory McIlroy's journey in golf is not just defined by his accomplishments on the course but also by the rivalries he has faced and the relationships he has forged along the way. From fierce competitors to trusted confidants, McIlroy's interactions with others have played a significant role in shaping his career and personal growth. As he continues to navigate the highs and lows of professional golf, McIlroy remains steadfast in his commitment to fostering meaningful connections and embracing the spirit of competition with grace and integrity.

8.1: Rory McIlroy: Competing Against Golf's Elite

Rory McIlroy's journey in professional golf has been defined by his relentless pursuit of excellence and his ability to compete against the sport's elite. From his early days as a prodigious talent to his current status as one of the game's most accomplished players, McIlroy's quest for greatness has seen him face off against some of golf's most formidable opponents on the biggest stages.

Rise to Prominence:

McIlroy burst onto the scene as a precocious young talent from Northern Ireland, showcasing a rare combination of power, precision, and poise on the golf course. His breakthrough victory at the 2011 U.S. Open, where he dominated the field to claim his first major

The Drive of Rory McIlroy

championship, announced his arrival as a force to be reckoned with in the world of golf.

Competing against the Legends:

Throughout his career, McIlroy has gone head-to-head with golfing legends such as Tiger Woods, Phil Mickelson, and Ernie Els. These battles have not only tested McIlroy's skills and resilience but have also provided him with invaluable learning experiences and opportunities for growth.

McIlroy's rivalry with Woods, in particular, has captured the imagination of golf fans around the world. From their memorable duels at major championships to their friendly banter on and off the course, McIlroy and Woods have pushed each other to new heights, raising the level of competition in the process.

Chasing major championships :

At the heart of McIlroy's quest for greatness lies his pursuit of major championships—the ultimate measure of success in professional golf. With four major titles to

The Drive of Rory McIlroy

his name, including victories at the U.S. Open, the Open Championship, the PGA Championship, and the Masters Tournament, McIlroy has cemented his place among the game's all-time greats.

McIlroy's quest for major glory has seen him face stiff competition from golf's elite players, including Jordan Spieth, Brooks Koepka, and Dustin Johnson. These battles on golf's grandest stages have tested McIlroy's mettle and determination, pushing him to dig deep and summon his best when it matters most.

Staying Competitive:

As McIlroy continues his pursuit of excellence, he remains focused on staying competitive against golf's elite. Whether he's teeing it up at major championships, World Golf Championships, or regular tour events, McIlroy approaches each tournament with the same level of intensity and determination, knowing that victory is never guaranteed in the highly competitive world of professional golf.

The Drive of Rory McIlroy

Rory McIlroy's journey in professional golf is a testament to his ability to compete against the sport's elite players with skill, grace, and determination. From his early battles with golfing legends to his quest for major championship glory, McIlroy has consistently risen to the occasion, showcasing the talent and tenacity that have made him one of the game's most beloved and respected figures. As he continues his pursuit of excellence, McIlroy remains steadfast in his commitment to competing against golf's elite while inspiring future generations of players to dream big and chase their own greatness on the golf course.

8.2: Friendships and Camaraderie on Tour

Beyond the intense competition and pursuit of victory on the golf course, Rory McIlroy has cultivated meaningful friendships and fostered a sense of camaraderie among his peers on the professional golf tour. Through shared experiences, mutual respect, and genuine camaraderie, McIlroy has forged lasting bonds with fellow players, creating a sense of community within the highly competitive world of golf.

The Drive of Rory McIlroy

The Bond of Shared Experiences:

As a professional golfer, McIlroy understands the unique challenges and pressures that come with competing at the highest level. Whether it's navigating difficult courses, contending with unpredictable weather conditions, or managing the demands of travel and competition, McIlroy and his fellow players share a common bond forged through their shared experiences on tour.

These shared experiences serve as the foundation for the friendships and camaraderie that McIlroy has built with his peers. From practising together on the driving range to competing alongside one another in tournaments, McIlroy cherishes the camaraderie that comes from being part of the close-knit golfing community.

Mutual Respect and Support:

Central to McIlroy's approach to building friendships on tour is a deep sense of mutual respect and support for his fellow players. Regardless of their competitive rivalry on

The Drive of Rory McIlroy

the course, McIlroy maintains a genuine admiration for the talent, dedication, and achievements of his peers.

Whether it's congratulating a rival on a well-played round, offering words of encouragement during a slump, or celebrating a friend's victory, McIlroy exemplifies the spirit of sportsmanship and camaraderie that define the golfing community. His genuine support for his fellow players transcends the boundaries of competition, fostering a sense of camaraderie that extends beyond the fairways and greens.

Off-Course Bonds:

Away from the pressures of competition, McIlroy enjoys building off-course friendships with his fellow players, bonding over shared interests and experiences. Whether it's enjoying a round of golf together during downtime, socialising at tour events, or simply spending time with friends and family, McIlroy values the connections he has forged with his peers outside of the competitive arena.

Moreover, McIlroy's friendships extend beyond his fellow players to include caddies, coaches, and other members of the golfing community. These relationships enrich McIlroy's experience on tour, providing him with a support network of trusted confidants and allies.

Rory McIlroy's approach to building friendships and fostering camaraderie on the golf course The course exemplifies the values of sportsmanship, mutual respect, and community that define the game of golf. Through shared experiences, genuine support, and off-course bonds, McIlroy has cultivated meaningful relationships with his peers, creating a sense of camaraderie that transcends the boundaries of competition. As he continues his journey in professional golf, McIlroy remains committed to nurturing these friendships and celebrating the camaraderie that makes the sport truly special.

8.3: Legacy and Impact on the Sport

Rory McIlroy's impact on the sport of golf extends far beyond his achievements on the course. Through his

The Drive of Rory McIlroy

remarkable talent, sportsmanship, and philanthropy, McIlroy has left an indelible mark on the game, shaping a legacy that will be celebrated for generations to come.

On-Course Achievements:

McIlroy's legacy in golf is built on a foundation of unparalleled success on the course. With four major championship titles, including victories at the U.S. Open, the Open Championship, the PGA Championship, and the Masters Tournament, McIlroy has cemented his place among the game's all-time greats.

His aggressive style of play, prodigious distance off the tee, and deft touch around the greens have captivated fans and fellow players alike, earning him admiration and respect throughout the golfing world. McIlroy's ability to rise to the occasion in the biggest moments, coupled with his consistency and longevity at the highest level of the sport, have solidified his status as a true icon of the game.

Off-Course Impact:

The Drive of Rory McIlroy

Beyond his accomplishments on the course, McIlroy's impact on the sport of golf extends to his off-course endeavours. As a global ambassador for the game, McIlroy has worked tirelessly to promote golf at all levels, from grassroots initiatives to elite competition.

Through his charitable foundation, McIlroy has made significant contributions to causes close to his heart, including children's health, education, and community development. His philanthropic efforts have touched the lives of countless individuals around the world, leaving a lasting legacy of generosity and compassion.

Moreover, McIlroy's influence extends beyond the golf course to the broader sports landscape. As a role model and ambassador for the game, McIlroy has inspired countless young athletes to pursue their dreams and strive for excellence in their chosen endeavours.

Legacy of Sportsmanship and Integrity:

Central to McIlroy's legacy in golf is his unwavering commitment to sportsmanship, integrity, and fair play. Throughout his career, McIlroy has conducted himself

The Drive of Rory McIlroy

with grace, humility, and respect for his fellow competitors, earning admiration and accolades for his conduct both on and off the course.

Whether in victory or defeat, McIlroy has exemplified the values of sportsmanship and integrity that are synonymous with the game of golf. His commitment to upholding the highest standards of conduct and professionalism has earned him the admiration and respect of fans, fellow players, and golf officials alike.

Rory McIlroy's legacy in the sport of golf is one of unparalleled achievement, impact, and influence. Through his remarkable talent, philanthropy, and commitment to sportsmanship, McIlroy has left an indelible mark on the game, shaping a legacy that will endure for generations to come. As he continues his journey in golf and beyond, McIlroy remains committed to making a positive difference in the world and inspiring others to reach their full potential, both on and off the course.

CHAPTER 9: THE FUTURE OF RORY MCILROY:

A Continuing Journey of Excellence and Impact

As Rory McIlroy continues his illustrious career in professional golf, the world eagerly anticipates what the future holds for this iconic athlete. With a legacy already etched in the annals of the sport, McIlroy's journey is poised to evolve, driven by a relentless pursuit of excellence, a commitment to philanthropy, and a desire to inspire future generations of golfers.

Quest for Major Championships:

At the forefront of McIlroy's aspirations is the pursuit of major championship glory. With four major titles already to his name, including victories at the U.S. Open, the Open Championship, the PGA Championship, and the Masters Tournament, McIlroy remains determined to add to his impressive tally of major victories.

The Drive of Rory McIlroy

The elusive quest for golf's most prestigious titles continues to fuel McIlroy's competitive fire, driving him to hone his skills, refine his game, and rise to the occasion on golf's grandest stages. With his talent, experience, and unwavering dedication, McIlroy is well-positioned to contend for major championships well into the future, solidifying his place among the game's all-time greats.

Impact Beyond the Fairways:

Beyond his pursuit of on-course success, McIlroy's impact extends to his off-course endeavours, where he uses his platform to effect positive change and make a difference in the world. Through his charitable foundation and philanthropic initiatives, McIlroy remains committed to supporting causes close to his heart, including children's health, education, and community development.

As McIlroy's influence continues to grow, so too does his capacity to effect meaningful change and inspire others to make a difference in their own communities. Whether through charitable giving, advocacy work, or mentorship programmes, McIlroy's impact transcends the boundaries

The Drive of Rory McIlroy

of sport, leaving a lasting legacy of compassion, generosity, and social responsibility.

Inspiring the Next Generation:

Central to McIlroy's vision for the future is his desire to inspire and empower the next generation of golfers to dream big, chase their goals, and reach their full potential. Through his actions on and off the course, McIlroy serves as a role model and mentor for aspiring young athletes, sharing his wisdom, experience, and passion for the game with those who look up to him.

By embodying the values of hard work, perseverance, and sportsmanship, McIlroy empowers young golfers to believe in themselves, overcome obstacles, and pursue their dreams with confidence and determination. As he continues his journey in golf and beyond, McIlroy remains committed to fostering a culture of excellence, inclusivity, and opportunity within the sport, ensuring that his legacy will endure for generations to come.

As Rory McIlroy looks to the future, his journey remains one of limitless potential, boundless opportunity, and enduring impact. With a commitment to excellence, a passion for philanthropy, and a dedication to inspiring others, McIlroy's legacy continues to evolve, shaping the future of golf and leaving an indelible mark on the world. As he embarks on the next chapter of his career, McIlroy's unwavering determination, humility, and grace will continue to inspire and uplift all those who have the privilege of witnessing his remarkable journey.

9.1: Charting a Course of Ambition and Aspiration

Rory McIlroy, with his unparalleled talent and relentless drive, has set his sights on a myriad of goals and aspirations that transcend the boundaries of the golf course. From major championship victories to philanthropic endeavours, McIlroy's vision for the future is shaped by a deep-seated ambition to make a meaningful impact on and off the fairways.

On-Course Ambitions:

The Drive of Rory McIlroy

At the pinnacle of McIlroy's aspirations lies the pursuit of major championship glory. With four major titles already in his illustrious career, McIlroy remains steadfast in his quest to add to his impressive tally and etch his name further into the annals of golfing history. His ultimate goal is to achieve the career Grand Slam, a feat that only a select few golfers have accomplished.

In addition to major championships, McIlroy is driven by a desire to reclaim the world number one ranking and solidify his status as one of the game's greatest players. With his prodigious talent, unwavering focus, and commitment to continuous improvement, McIlroy is poised to remain a dominant force on the PGA Tour and the international golf circuit for years to come.

Off-Course Aspirations:

Beyond his on-course pursuits, McIlroy's aspirations extend to making a meaningful impact off the golf course. Through his charitable foundation and philanthropic initiatives, McIlroy is dedicated to supporting causes that are close to his heart, including children's health, education, and community development.

The Drive of Rory McIlroy

McIlroy's goal is to leverage his platform and influence to effect positive change and improve the lives of others. Whether through fundraising efforts, advocacy work, or hands-on involvement in charitable projects, McIlroy is committed to making a difference in the world and leaving a lasting legacy of compassion, generosity, and social responsibility.

Personal Growth and Development:

In addition to his professional and philanthropic goals, McIlroy is committed to personal growth and development both on and off the golf course. He seeks to continually refine his skills, expand his knowledge, and evolve as a person and as an athlete.

McIlroy's aspirations for personal growth extend to his relationships, his family life, and his overall well-being. He strives to strike a balance between his professional commitments and his personal life, nurturing meaningful connections with loved ones and finding fulfilment beyond the confines of competition.

The Drive of Rory McIlroy

Rory McIlroy's journey is fueled by a relentless pursuit of excellence, a commitment to making a difference, and a desire to grow and evolve as both an athlete and a human being. With his eyes set firmly on the future, McIlroy's goals and aspirations serve as a guiding light, illuminating a path of ambition, achievement, and impact that will continue to inspire and uplift all those who follow his remarkable journey.

9.2: Continuing to Push the Boundaries and Redefining Greatness

Rory McIlroy's journey in professional golf has been defined by his relentless pursuit of excellence and his willingness to push the boundaries of what is possible in the sport. As he continues to evolve as a player and a person, McIlroy remains committed to challenging himself, breaking barriers, and redefining the limits of his potential on and off the golf course.

Pushing the Limits of Performance

The Drive of Rory McIlroy

At the heart of McIlroy's approach to the game is a constant quest to push the boundaries of performance and unlock new levels of achievement. Whether it's through technical innovation, mental resilience, or physical conditioning, McIlroy is always seeking ways to elevate his game and stay at the forefront of his sport.

McIlroy's commitment to pushing the limits of performance is evident in his relentless pursuit of major championship victories and world number one rankings. With his prodigious talent, unwavering work ethic, and insatiable hunger for success, McIlroy continues to set new standards of excellence and inspire awe with his feats on the golf course.

Embracing Innovation and Adaptation:

As the game of golf evolves, so too does McIlroy's approach to the sport. He embraces innovation and adaptation, constantly refining his technique, strategy, and equipment to stay ahead of the curve and remain competitive in an ever-changing landscape.

The Drive of Rory McIlroy

From adopting new technologies and training methods to fine-tuning his swing and short game, McIlroy is not afraid to experiment and push the boundaries of convention in his quest for improvement. His willingness to embrace change and evolve with the times has been instrumental in his continued success and longevity in the sport.

Breaking Barriers and Inspiring Others:

Beyond his own achievements, McIlroy is driven by a desire to break down barriers and inspire others to reach their full potential. Whether it's through his philanthropic endeavours, his advocacy work, or his role as a mentor and ambassador for the game, McIlroy strives to make a positive impact on the world and leave a lasting legacy of empowerment and inspiration.

By pushing the boundaries of what is possible in golf and in life, McIlroy serves as a beacon of hope and possibility for aspiring athletes, dreamers, and achievers around the world. His journey is a testament to the power of perseverance, passion, and determination to overcome obstacles and achieve greatness against all odds.

Rory McIlroy's journey is one of constant evolution, innovation, and inspiration. As he continues to push the boundaries of what is possible in professional golf and beyond, McIlroy serves as a role model and a trailblazer, showing us that with dedication, courage, and vision, anything is possible. As he embarks on the next chapter of his remarkable journey, McIlroy's unwavering commitment to pushing the limits of performance and breaking down barriers will continue to inspire and uplift all those who have the privilege of witnessing his extraordinary feats.

9.3: Legacy Beyond the Fairways

Rory McIlroy's impact extends far beyond the boundaries of the golf course, shaping a legacy that transcends the sport itself. Through his philanthropy, advocacy, and commitment to making a difference, McIlroy has left an indelible mark on the world, inspiring others to dream big, give back, and strive for excellence in all aspects of life.

The Drive of Rory McIlroy

Philanthropic Endeavours:

At the core of McIlroy's legacy is his dedication to philanthropy and giving back to those in need. Through his charitable foundation, McIlroy has supported a wide range of causes, including children's health, education, and community development.

From funding medical research and providing resources for underserved communities to supporting youth programmes and educational initiatives, McIlroy's philanthropic efforts have touched the lives of countless individuals around the world, leaving a lasting impact that extends far beyond the fairways.

Advocacy and Social Responsibility:

In addition to his philanthropic endeavours, McIlroy is a passionate advocate for social change and environmental sustainability. He uses his platform and influence to raise awareness about important issues, from climate change and conservation to equality and social justice.

The Drive of Rory McIlroy

McIlroy's advocacy work is driven by a deep sense of social responsibility and a belief in the power of individuals to make a positive difference in the world. Whether speaking out on behalf of marginalised communities, supporting environmental initiatives, or championing causes close to his heart, McIlroy remains committed to using his voice for good and inspiring others to do the same.

Inspiring the Next Generation:

Central to McIlroy's legacy is his role as a mentor and inspiration for the next generation of athletes, leaders, and changemakers. Through his actions on and off the golf course, McIlroy empowers young people to dream big, set goals, and pursue their passions with determination and resilience.

Whether through his philanthropic work, his advocacy efforts, or his unwavering commitment to excellence, McIlroy serves as a role model and mentor for aspiring individuals around the world. His journey is a testament to the power of perseverance, hard work, and belief in oneself to overcome obstacles and achieve greatness.

The Drive of Rory McIlroy

Rory McIlroy's legacy extends far beyond the fairways, encompassing a legacy of philanthropy, advocacy, and inspiration that will endure for generations to come. Through his unwavering commitment to making a difference in the world, McIlroy has left an indelible mark on the lives of countless individuals, inspiring others to follow in his footsteps and strive for excellence in all that they do. As he continues his journey, McIlroy's legacy will serve as a beacon of hope and inspiration for generations to come, reminding us all of the power of compassion, courage, and commitment to create a better world for future generations.

CHAPTER 10: REFLECTIONS AND LESSONS :

Reflections on a Journey of Success and Lessons Learned

As Rory McIlroy reflects on his journey in professional golf, he recognises the profound impact it has had on his life and the invaluable lessons it has taught him along the way. From the highs of major championship victories to the challenges of setbacks and adversity, McIlroy's reflections offer insights into the complexities of success and the enduring power of resilience, determination, and growth.

Lessons from Success:

McIlroy's journey is punctuated by moments of triumph and success, each one offering valuable lessons and insights into the nature of achievement. Whether it's winning his first major championship or reclaiming the world number one ranking, McIlroy understands the importance of hard work, dedication, and belief in oneself in the pursuit of greatness.

The Drive of Rory McIlroy

Through his successes, McIlroy has learned the importance of staying grounded, remaining humble, and never taking anything for granted. He recognises that success is not just about winning trophies or accolades but about the journey itself and the lessons learned along the way.

Navigating Setbacks and Adversity:

Despite his many triumphs, McIlroy's journey has also been marked by setbacks and challenges, from injuries and slumps in form to disappointments on the biggest stages. Through these experiences, McIlroy has learned the importance of resilience, perseverance, and mental toughness in overcoming adversity and bouncing back stronger than ever.

McIlroy's ability to weather the storms of disappointment and adversity has taught him valuable lessons about the importance of resilience and perseverance in the face of adversity. He understands that setbacks are an inevitable part of life and that true strength lies in how we respond to them.

The Drive of Rory McIlroy

Growth and Evolution:

As McIlroy reflects on his journey, he recognises the importance of growth, evolution, and continuous improvement in both his game and his personal life. He understands that success is not static but rather a journey of growth and self-discovery that requires constant adaptation and reinvention.

McIlroy's willingness to embrace change, learn from his mistakes, and evolve as both a player and a person has been instrumental in his continued success and longevity in the sport. He understands that growth requires stepping out of one's comfort zone, taking risks, and embracing new challenges with courage and determination.

Rory McIlroy's reflections offer a window into the lessons learned from a lifetime of dedication, perseverance, and passion for the game of golf. From the highs of success to the lows of adversity, McIlroy's journey is a testament to the enduring power of resilience, determination, and growth in the pursuit of excellence. As he continues to evolve and grow, McIlroy remains committed to embracing the lessons of his journey and inspiring others to do the same, reminding us all of the transformative power of reflection, resilience, and self-discovery in the pursuit of our dreams.

10.1: Inspirational Insights for Golfers and Fans Alike

Rory McIlroy's journey in professional golf is filled with inspirational insights and valuable lessons that resonate with golfers and fans alike. From his unwavering determination to his commitment to excellence, McIlroy's journey offers a wealth of wisdom and inspiration for those seeking to excel in golf and in life.

1. Pursue your passion with purpose.

McIlroy's passion for golf has been evident since childhood, driving him to pursue his dreams with unwavering determination and commitment. His journey serves as a reminder that true success comes from following your passion with purpose, dedicating yourself wholeheartedly to your craft, and never losing sight of your goals.

2. Embrace challenges as opportunities.

Throughout his career, McIlroy has faced his fair share of challenges, from injuries and setbacks to the pressures of competition on the biggest stages. Instead of allowing adversity to derail him, McIlroy has embraced challenges as opportunities for growth, learning, and self-improvement. His journey teaches us that resilience, perseverance, and a positive mindset are essential qualities for overcoming obstacles and achieving success.

3. Stay humble in victory and defeat.

Despite his numerous accomplishments and accolades, McIlroy remains humble and grounded, both in victory and defeat. He understands that success is fleeting and that humility is essential for maintaining perspective and staying true to oneself. McIlroy's humility serves as a reminder that true greatness is measured not only by what we achieve but by how we conduct ourselves along the way.

4. Give back and make a difference.

McIlroy's commitment to philanthropy and giving back to those in need exemplifies the power of using one's platform for good. He understands that success is not just about personal achievement but about making a positive impact on the world and leaving a lasting legacy of compassion, generosity, and social responsibility. McIlroy's journey inspires us to look beyond ourselves and find ways to give back to our communities and make a difference in the lives of others.

5. Never stop learning and growing.

Throughout his career, McIlroy has demonstrated a willingness to learn, adapt, and evolve as both a player and a person. He understands that growth requires stepping out of one's comfort zone, taking risks, and embracing new challenges with courage and determination. McIlroy's journey reminds us that the pursuit of excellence is a lifelong journey of learning, growth, and self-discovery.

The Drive of Rory McIlroy

Rory McIlroy's journey in professional golf offers a wealth of inspirational insights and valuable lessons for golfers and fans alike. From his unwavering passion and determination to his commitment to giving back and making a difference, McIlroy's journey serves as a source of inspiration and motivation for all who aspire to achieve their dreams and make a positive impact on the world. As we navigate our own journeys, let us draw inspiration from McIlroy's example and strive to pursue our passions with purpose, embrace challenges as opportunities for growth, stay humble in victory and defeat, give back to our communities, and never stop learning and growing along the way.

The Drive of Rory McIlroy

CONCLUSION:

In the captivating pages of The Drive of Rory McIlroy: A Golfing Legend, readers have embarked on a journey through the extraordinary life and career of one of golf's most iconic figures. From his humble beginnings in Northern Ireland to his ascension to the pinnacle of the sport, Rory McIlroy's story is one of relentless determination, unwavering passion, and unparalleled success.

As the final chapter of this compelling narrative draws to a close, it is clear that McIlroy's drive for excellence extends far beyond the fairways and greens. Through his remarkable talent, unwavering work ethic, and commitment to making a difference, McIlroy has not only left an indelible mark on the world of golf but has also inspired countless individuals to dream big, pursue their passions, and strive for greatness in all aspects of life.

In the pages of this book, readers have been treated to a wealth of insights, lessons, and inspiration gleaned from McIlroy's remarkable journey. From the highs of major championship victories to the challenges of setbacks and

The Drive of Rory McIlroy

adversity, McIlroy's story serves as a testament to the enduring power of resilience, determination, and self-belief in the pursuit of one's dreams.

As readers reflect on the pages of The Drive of Rory McIlroy: A Golfing Legend, they are reminded that greatness is not defined solely by victories and accolades but by the character, integrity, and impact one leaves behind. Through his philanthropic endeavours, advocacy work, and unwavering commitment to excellence, McIlroy has left a legacy that extends far beyond the confines of the golf course, inspiring generations to come to strive for excellence, make a difference, and leave their mark on the world.

The Drive of Rory McIlroy: A Golfing Legend stands as a tribute to the enduring legacy of one of golf's greatest champions. As readers turn the final page, they are left with a profound sense of admiration, inspiration, and gratitude for the remarkable journey of a true sporting legend.

www.ingramcontent.com/pod-product-compliance
Lightning Source LLC
Chambersburg PA
CBHW050108230526
45470CB00004B/1731